INFECTIOUS DISEASE DEATHS IN SOUTH AUSTRALIA

Donald Bradman

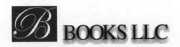

BOOKS LLC

Publication Data:

Title: Infectious Disease Deaths in South Australia

Subtitle: Donald Bradman

Published by: Books LLC, Memphis, Tennessee, USA in 2010

Copyright (chapters): http://creativecommons.org/licenses/by-sa/3.0

Online edition: http://booksllc.net/?q=Category:Infectious_disease_deaths_in_South_Australia

Contact the publisher: http://booksllc.net/contactus.cfm

CONTENTS

Introduction

The online edition of this book is at http://booksllc.net/?q=Category:Infectious%
5Fdisease%5Fdeaths%5Fin%5FSouth%5FAustralia. It's hyperlinked and may be
updated. Where we have recommended related pages, you can read them at
http://booksllc.net/?q= followed by the page's title. Most entries in the book's index also have a dedicated page at http://booksllc.net/?q= followed by the index entry.

Each chapter in this book ends with a URL to a hyperlinked online version. Use the
online version to access related pages, websites, footnote URLs. You can click the
history tab on the online version to see a list of the chapter's contributors. While we
have included photo captions in the book, due to copyright restrictions you can only
view the photos online. You also need to go to the online edition to view some formula
symbols.

The online version of this book is part of Wikipedia, a multilingual, web-based
encyclopedia.

Wikipedia is written collaboratively. Since its creation in 2001, Wikipedia has grown
rapidly into one of the largest reference web sites, attracting nearly 68 million visitors
monthly. There are more than 91,000 active contributors working on more than 15

million articles in more than 270 languages. Every day, hundreds of thousands of active from around the world collectively make tens of thousands of edits and create thousands of new articles.

After a long process of discussion, debate, and argument, articles gradually take on a neutral point of view reached through consensus. Additional editors expand and contribute to articles and strive to achieve balance and comprehensive coverage. Wikipedia's intent is to cover existing knowledge which is verifiable from other sources. The ideal Wikipedia article is well-written, balanced, neutral, and encyclopedic, containing comprehensive, notable, verifiable knowledge.

Wikipedia is open to a large contributor base, drawing a large number of editors from diverse backgrounds. This allows Wikipedia to significantly reduce regional and cultural bias found in many other publications, and makes it very difficult for any group to censor and impose bias. A large, diverse editor base also provides access and breadth on subject matter that is otherwise inaccessible or little documented.

Think you can improve the book? If so, simply go to the online version and suggest changes. If accepted, your additions could appear in the next edition!

DONALD BRADMAN

- Personal information
- Full name: Donald George Bradman
- Born: 27 August 1908(1908-08-27) Cootamundra, New South Wales, Australia
- Died: 25 February 2001 (aged 92) Kensington Park, South Australia, Australia
- Nickname: The Don, The Boy from Bowral, Braddles
- Height: 1.70 m (5 ft 7 in)
- Batting style: Right-handed
- Bowling style: Right-arm leg break
- Role: Batsman
- International information
- National side: Australia
- Test debut (cap 124): 30 November 1928 v England
- Last Test: 18 August 1948 v England
- Domestic team information
- Years: Team
- 1927 34: New South Wales
- 1935 49: South Australia
- Career statistics
- Competition: Tests: FC

- Matches: 52: 234
- Runs scored: 6,996: 28,067
- Batting average: 99.94: 95.14
- 100s/50s: 29/13: 117/69
- Top score: 334: 452*
- Balls bowled: 160: 2114
- Wickets: 2: 36
- Bowling average: 36.00: 37.97
- 5 wickets in innings: 0: 0
- 10 wickets in match: 0: 0
- Best bowling: 1/8: 3/35
- Catches/stumpings: 32/ : 131/1
- Source: Cricinfo, 16 August 2007

Sir Donald George Bradman, AC (27 August 1908 25 February 2001), often referred to as **The Don**, was an Australian cricketer, widely acknowledged as the greatest batsman of all time.[1] Bradman's career Test batting average of 99.94 has been claimed to be statistically the greatest achievement in any major sport.[2]

The story that the young Bradman practised alone with a cricket stump and a golf ball is part of Australian folklore.[3] Bradman's meteoric rise from bush cricket to the Australian Test team took just over two years. Before his 22nd birthday, he had set many records for high scoring, some of which still stand, and became Australia's sporting idol at the height of the Great Depression.

During a 20-year playing career, Bradman consistently scored at a level that made him, in the words of former Australia captain Bill Woodfull, "worth three batsmen to Australia".[4] A controversial set of tactics, known as Bodyline, was specifically devised by the England team to curb his scoring. As a captain and administrator Bradman was committed to attacking, entertaining cricket; he drew spectators in record numbers. He hated the constant adulation, however, and it affected how he dealt with others. The focus of attention on his individual performances strained relationships with some team-mates, administrators and journalists, who thought him aloof and wary.[5] Following an enforced hiatus, due to the Second World War, he made a dramatic comeback, captaining an Australian team known as "The Invincibles" on a record-breaking unbeaten tour of England.

A complex, highly driven man, not given to close personal relationships,[6] Bradman retained a pre-eminent position in the game by acting as an administrator, selector and writer for three decades following his retirement. Even after he became reclusive in his declining years his opinion was highly sought, and his status as a national icon was still recognised more than 50 years after his retirement as a Test player, in 2001, the Australian Prime Minister John Howard called him the "greatest living Australian".[7] Bradman's image has appeared on postage stamps and coins, and he was the first living Australian to have a museum dedicated to his life. On the centenary of his birth, 27

August 2008, the Royal Australian Mint issued a $5 commemorative gold coin with his image.[8]

On 19 November 2009, Sir Don Bradman was inducted into the ICC Cricket Hall of Fame.[9]

Early years

Online image: Bradman's birthplace at Cootamundra is now a museum.

Donald Bradman was the youngest son of George and Emily (née Whatman) Bradman, and was born on 27 August 1908 at Cootamundra, New South Wales (NSW).[10] He had a brother, Victor, and three sisters Islet, Lilian and Elizabeth May.[10] When Bradman was about two-and-a-half years old, his parents moved to Bowral in the NSW Southern Highlands.[10]

Bradman practised batting incessantly during his youth. He invented his own solo cricket game, using a cricket stump for a bat, and a golf ball.[11] A water tank, mounted on a curved brick stand, stood on a paved area behind the family home. When hit into the curved brick facing of the stand, the ball rebounded at high speed and varying angles and Bradman would attempt to hit it again. This form of practice developed his timing and reactions to a high degree.[12] In more formal cricket, he hit his first century at the age of 12, playing for Bowral Public School against Mittagong High School.[13]

Bush cricketer

In 1920 21, Bradman acted as scorer for the local Bowral team, captained by his uncle George Whatman. In October 1920, he filled in when the team was one man short, scoring 37 not out and 29 not out on debut. During the season, Bradman's father took him to the Sydney Cricket Ground (SCG) to watch the fifth Ashes Test match. On that day, Bradman formed an ambition. "I shall never be satisfied", he told his father, "until I play on this ground".[14] Bradman left school in 1922 and went to work for a local real estate agent who encouraged his sporting pursuits by giving him time off when necessary. He gave up cricket in favour of tennis for two years, but resumed playing cricket in 1925 26.[15]

Bradman became a regular selection for the Bowral team; several outstanding performances earned him the attention of the Sydney daily press. Competing on matting-over-concrete pitches, Bowral played other rural towns in the Berrima District competition. Against Wingello, a team that included the future Test bowler Bill O'Reilly, Bradman made 234.[4][16] In the competition final against Moss Vale, which extended over five consecutive Saturdays, Bradman scored 320 not out.[13] During the following Australian winter (1926), an ageing Australian team lost The Ashes in England, and a number of Test players retired.[17] The New South Wales Cricket

Association began a hunt for new talent. Mindful of Bradman's big scores for Bowral, the association wrote to him, requesting his attendance at a practice session in Sydney. He was subsequently chosen for the "Country Week" tournaments at both cricket and tennis, to be played during separate weeks. His boss presented him with an ultimatum: he could have only one week away from work, and therefore had to choose between the two sports.[15] He chose cricket. Bradman's performances during Country Week resulted in an invitation to play grade cricket in Sydney for St George in the 1926 27 season. He scored 110 on his debut, making his first century on a turf wicket.[18] On 1 January 1927, he turned out for the NSW second team. For the remainder of the season, Bradman travelled the 130 kilometres (81 mi) from Bowral to Sydney every Saturday to play for St George.[16]

First-class debut

Online image: Bradman in 1928

The next season continued the rapid rise of the "Boy from Bowral".[13] Selected to replace the unfit Archie Jackson in the NSW team, Bradman made his first-class debut at the Adelaide Oval, aged 19. He secured the achievement of a hundred on debut, with an innings of 118 featuring what soon became his trademarks fast footwork, calm confidence and rapid scoring.[19] In the final match of the season, he made his first century at the SCG, against the Sheffield Shield champions Victoria. Despite his potential, Bradman was not chosen for the Australian second team to tour New Zealand.[20]

Bradman decided that his chances for Test selection would be improved by moving to Sydney for the 1928 29 season, when England were to tour in defence of the Ashes. Initially, he continued working in real estate, but later took a promotions job with the sporting goods retailer Mick Simmons Ltd. In the first match of the Sheffield Shield season, he scored a century in each innings against Queensland. He followed this with scores of 87 and 132 not out against the England touring team, and was rewarded with selection for the first Test, to be played at Brisbane.[15]

Test career

Online image: Bradman is chaired off the ground by his opponents after scoring 452.

Playing in only his tenth first-class match, Bradman, nicknamed "Braddles" by his teammates,[21] found his initial Test a harsh learning experience. Caught on a sticky wicket, Australia were all out for 66 in the second innings and lost by 675 runs (still a Test record).[22] Following scores of 18 and 1, the selectors dropped Bradman to twelfth man for the Second Test. An injury to Bill Ponsford early in the match required Bradman to field as substitute while England amassed 636, following their 863 runs in the First Test. RS Whitington wrote, "... he had scored only nineteen himself and these experiences appear to have provided him with food for thought".[23] Recalled for the Third Test at the Melbourne Cricket Ground, Bradman scored 79 and 112 to become the youngest player to make a Test century,[24] although the match was still lost. Another loss followed in the Fourth Test. Bradman reached 58 in the second innings and appeared set to guide the team to victory when he was run out.[25] It was to be the only run out of his Test career. The losing margin was just 12 runs.[26]

Online image: Bradman with his Wm. Sykes bat, in the early 1930s. The "Don Bradman Autograph" bat is still manufactured today by Sykes' successor company, Slazenger.

The improving Australians did manage to win the Fifth and final Test. Bradman top-scored with 123 in the first innings, and was at the wicket in the second innings when his captain Jack Ryder hit the winning runs. Bradman completed the season with 1,690 first-class runs, averaging 93.88,[27] and his first multiple century in a Sheffield Shield match, 340 not out against Victoria, set a new ground record for the SCG.[28] Bradman averaged 113.28 in 1929 30.[27] In a trial match to select the team that would tour England, he was last man out in the first innings for 124. As his team followed on, the skipper Bill Woodfull asked Bradman to keep the pads on and open the second innings. By the end of play, he was 205 not out, on his way to 225. Against Queensland at the SCG, Bradman set a world record for first-class cricket by scoring 452 not out; he made his runs in only 415 minutes.[15] Not long after the feat, he recalled:

On 434 ..., I had a curious intuition ... I seemed to sense that the ball would be a short-pitched one on the leg-stump, and I could almost feel myself getting ready to make my shot before the ball was delivered. Sure enough, it pitched exactly where I had anticipated, and, hooking it to the square-leg boundary, I established the only record upon which I had set my heart.[29]

Although he was an obvious selection to tour England, Bradman's unorthodox style raised doubts that he could succeed on the slower English pitches. Percy Fender wrote:[30]

... he will always be in the category of the brilliant, if unsound, ones. Promise there is in Bradman in plenty, though watching him does not inspire one with any confidence that he desires to take the only course which will lead him to a fulfilment of that promise. He makes a mistake, then makes it again and again; he does not correct it, or look as if he were trying to do so. He seems to live for the exuberance of the moment.

The encomiums were not confined to his batting gifts; nor did the criticism extend to his character. "Australia has unearthed a champion," raved former Australian Test great Clem Hill, "self-taught, with natural ability. But most important of all, with his heart in the right place."[29] Selector Dick Jones weighed in with the observation that it was "good to watch him talking to an old player, listening attentively to everything that is said and then replying with a modest 'thank you'."[29]

1930 tour of England

England were favourites to win the 1930 Ashes series,[31] and if the Australians were to exceed expectations, their young batsmen, Bradman and Jackson, needed to prosper. With his elegant batting technique, Jackson appeared the brighter prospect of the pair.[32] However, Bradman began the tour with 236 at Worcester and went on to score 1,000 first-class runs by the end of May, the fifth player (and first Australian) to achieve this rare feat.[33] In his first Test appearance in England, Bradman hit 131 in the second innings but England won the match. His batting reached a new level in the Second Test at Lord's where he scored 254 as Australia won and levelled the series. Later in life, Bradman rated this the best innings of his career as, "practically without exception every ball went where it was intended to go".[34] *Wisden* noted his fast footwork and how he hit the ball "all round the wicket with power and accuracy", as well as faultless concentration in keeping the ball on the ground.[35]

In terms of runs scored, this performance was soon surpassed. In the Third Test, at Leeds, Bradman scored a century before lunch on the first day of the Test match to equal the performances of Victor Trumper and Charlie Macartney.[36] In the afternoon, Bradman added another century between lunch and tea, before finishing the day on 309 not out. He remains the only Test player to pass 300 in one day's play.[37] His eventual score of 334 was a world-record, exceeding the previous mark of 325 by Andy Sandham.[38] Bradman dominated the Australian innings; the second-highest tally was 77 by Alan Kippax. Businessman Arthur Whitelaw later presented Bradman with a cheque for $1,000 in appreciation of his achievement.[39] The match ended in anti-climax as poor weather prevented a result, as it had done in the Fourth Test.

Online image: Bradman (second from the right, middle row) with the 1930 team

In the deciding Test at The Oval, England made 405. During an innings stretching over three days due to intermittent rain, Bradman made yet another multiple century, this time 232, which helped give Australia a big lead of 290 runs. In a crucial partnership with Archie Jackson, Bradman battled through a difficult session when England fast bowler Harold Larwood bowled short on a pitch enlivened by the rain. *Wisden* gave this period of play only a passing mention:[40]

On the Wednesday morning the ball flew about a good deal, both batsmen frequently being hit on the body ... on more than one occasion each player cocked the ball up dangerously but always, as it happened, just wide of the fieldsmen.

A number of English players and commentators noted Bradman's discomfort in playing the short, rising delivery.[4] The revelation came too late for this particular match, but was to have immense significance in the next Ashes series. Australia won the match by an innings and regained the Ashes. The victory made an impact in Australia. With the economy sliding toward depression and unemployment rapidly rising, the country found solace in sporting triumph. The story of a self-taught 22-year-old from the bush who set a series of records against the old rival made Bradman a national hero.[41] The statistics Bradman achieved on the tour, and in the Test matches in particular, broke records for the day and some have stood the test of time. In all, Bradman scored 974 runs at an average of 139.14 during the Test series, with four centuries, including two double hundreds and a triple.[42] As of 2008, no-one has matched or exceeded 974 runs or three double centuries in one Test series; the record of 974 runs exceeds the second-best performance by 69 runs and was achieved in two fewer innings.[43] Bradman's first-class tally, 2,960 runs (at an average of 98.66 with 10 centuries), was another enduring record: the most by any overseas batsman on a tour of England.[44]

On the tour, the dynamic nature of Bradman's batting contrasted sharply with his quiet, solitary off-field demeanour. He was described as aloof from his teammates and he did not offer to buy them a round of drinks, let alone share the money given to him by Whitelaw.[6] Bradman spent a lot of his free time alone, writing, as he had sold the rights to a book. On his return to Australia, Bradman was surprised by the intensity of his reception; he became a "reluctant hero".[6] Mick Simmons wanted to cash in on their employee's newly won fame. They asked Bradman to leave his teammates and attend official receptions they organised in Adelaide, Melbourne, Goulburn, his hometown Bowral and Sydney, where he received a brand new custom-built Chevrolet. At each stop, Bradman received a level of adulation that "embarrassed" him. This focus on individual accomplishment, in a team game, "... permanently damaged relationships with his contemporaries".[6] Commenting on Australia's victory, the team's vice-captain Vic Richardson said, "... we could have played any team without Bradman, but we could not have played the blind school without Clarrie Grimmett".[45]

Reluctant hero

In 1930 31, against the first West Indian side to visit Australia, Bradman's scoring was more sedate than in England although he did make 223 in 297 minutes in the Third Test at Brisbane and 152 in 154 minutes in the following Test at Melbourne.[46] However, he scored quickly in a very successful sequence of innings against the South Africans in the Australian summer of 1931 32. For NSW against the tourists, he made 30, 135 and 219. In the Test matches, he scored 226 (277 minutes), 112 (155 minutes), 2 and 167 (183 minutes); his 299 not out in the Fourth Test, at Adelaide, set a new record for the highest score in a Test in Australia.[47][48] Australia won nine of the ten Tests played over the two series.

At this point, Bradman had played 15 Test matches since the beginning of 1930, scoring 2,227 runs at an average of 131.[49] He had played 18 innings, scoring 10 centuries, six of which had extended beyond 200.[49] His overall scoring rate was 42 runs per hour,[50] with 856 (or 38.5% of his tally) scored in boundaries.[49] Significantly, he had not hit a six,[49] which typified Bradman's attitude: if he hit the ball along the ground, then it could not be caught. During this phase of his career, his youth and natural fitness allowed him to adopt a "machine-like" approach to batting. The South African fast bowler Sandy Bell described bowling to him as, "heart-breaking ... with his sort of cynical grin, which rather reminds one of the Sphinx ... he never seems to perspire".[51]

Online image: Hundreds of onlookers gather as the Bradmans leave the church after their wedding ceremony in 1932.

Between these two seasons, Bradman seriously contemplated playing professional cricket in England with the Lancashire League club Accrington, a move that according to the rules of the day, would have ended his Test career.[15] A consortium of three Sydney businesses offered an alternative. They devised a two-year contract whereby Bradman wrote for Associated Newspapers, broadcast on Radio 2UE and promoted the menswear retailing chain FJ Palmer and Son.[15] However, the contract increased Bradman's dependence on his public profile, making it more difficult to maintain the privacy that he ardently desired.[51]

Bradman's chaotic wedding to Jessie Menzies in April 1932 epitomised these new and unwelcome intrusions into his private life. The church "was under siege all throughout the day ... uninvited guests stood on chairs and pews to get a better view"; police erected barriers that were broken down and many of those invited could not get a seat.[51] Just weeks later, Bradman joined a private team organised by Arthur Mailey to tour the United States and Canada. He travelled with his wife, and the couple treated the trip as a honeymoon. Playing 51 games in 75 days, Bradman scored 3,779 runs at 102.1, with 18 centuries. Although the standard of play was not high, the effects of the amount of cricket Bradman had played in the three years previous, together with the strains of his celebrity status, began to show on his return home.[52]

Bodyline

See also: Bodyline

As long as Australia has Bradman she will be invincible ... It is almost time to request a legal limit on the number of runs Bradman should be allowed to make.

News Chronicle, London[53]

Within the Marylebone Cricket Club (MCC), which administered English cricket at the time, few voices were more influential than "Plum" Warner's, who, when considering England's response to Bradman, wrote that it "must evolve a new type of bowler and develop fresh ideas and strange tactics to curb his almost uncanny skill". To that end, Warner orchestrated the appointment of Douglas Jardine as England captain in 1931, as a prelude to Jardine leading the 1932 33 tour to Australia, with Warner as team manager.[54] Remembering that Bradman had struggled against bouncers during his 232 at The Oval in 1930, Jardine decided to combine traditional leg theory with short-pitched bowling to combat Bradman. He settled on the Nottinghamshire fast bowlers Harold Larwood and Bill Voce as the spearheads for his tactics. In support, the England selectors chose another three pacemen for the squad. The unusually high number of fast bowlers caused a lot of comment in both countries and roused Bradman's own suspicions.[13]

Bradman had other problems to deal with at this time; among these were bouts of illness from an undiagnosed malaise which had begun during the tour of North America,[55] and that the Australian Board of Control had initially refused permission for him to write a column for the *Sydney Sun*.[55] Bradman, who had signed a two-year contract with the newspaper, threatened to withdraw from cricket to honour his contract when the board denied him permission to write; eventually, the paper released Bradman from the contract, in a victory for the Board.[55] In three first-class games against England before the Tests, Bradman averaged just 17.16 in 6 innings.[56] Jardine decided to give the new tactics a trial in only one game, a fixture against an Australian XI at Melbourne. In this match, Bradman faced the leg theory and later warned local administrators that trouble was brewing if it continued.[57] He withdrew from the First Test at the Sydney Cricket Ground amid rumours that he had suffered a nervous breakdown. Despite his absence, England employed what were already becoming known as the Bodyline tactics against the Australian batsmen and won an ill-tempered match.[15]

Online image: The famous duck: Bradman bowled by Bowes at the MCG, in front of a world record crowd assembled to see Bradman defeat Bodyline

The public clamoured for the return of Bradman to defeat Bodyline: "he was the batsman who could conquer this cankerous bowling ... 'Bradmania', amounting almost to religious fervour, demanded his return".[58] Recovered from his indisposition, Bradman returned to the side in Alan Kippax's position. A world record crowd of 63,993 at the MCG saw Bradman come to the crease on the first day of the Second Test with the score at 2/67. A standing ovation ensued that delayed play for several minutes.[59] Bradman anticipated receiving a bouncer as his first ball and, as the bowler delivered, he moved across his stumps to play the hook shot. The ball failed to rise and Bradman dragged it onto his stumps; the first-ball duck was his first in a Test. The crowd fell into stunned silence as he walked off. However, Australia took a first innings lead in the match, and another record crowd on 2 January 1933 watched Bradman hit a counter-attacking second innings century. His unbeaten 103 (from 146 balls) in a team total of 191 helped set England a target of 251 to win. Bill O'Reilly and Bert Ironmonger bowled Australia to a series-levelling victory amid hopes that Bodyline was beaten.[60]

The Third Test at the Adelaide Oval proved pivotal. There were angry crowd scenes after the Australian captain Bill Woodfull and wicket-keeper Bert Oldfield were hit by bouncers. An apologetic Plum Warner entered the Australian dressing room and was rebuked by Woodfull. Wooodfull's remarks (that "...there are 2 teams out there and only one of them is playing cricket") were leaked to the press, and Warner and others attributed this to Fingleton, however for many years (even after Fingleton's death) a bitter war of accusation passed between Fingleton and Bradman as to who was the real source of the leak. In a cable to the MCC, the Australian Board of Control repeated the allegation of poor sportsmanship directed at Warner by Woodfull.[61] With the support of the MCC, England continued with Bodyline despite Australian protests. The tourists won the last three Tests convincingly and regained the Ashes. Bradman caused controversy with his own tactics. Always seeking to score, and with the leg side packed with fielders, he often backed away and hit the ball into the vacant half of the outfield with unorthodox shots reminiscent of tennis or golf.[62] This brought him 396 runs (at 56.57) for the series and plaudits for attempting to find a solution to Bodyline, although his series average was just 57% of his career mean. Jack Fingleton was in no doubt that Bradman's game altered irrevocably as a consequence of Bodyline, writing:[63]

Bodyline was specially prepared, nurtured for and expended on him and, in consequence, his technique underwent a change quicker than might have been the case with the passage of time. Bodyline plucked something vibrant from his art.

The constant glare of celebrity and the tribulations of the season forced Bradman to reappraise his life outside the game and to seek a career away from his cricketing fame.[64] Harry Hodgetts, a South Australian delegate to the Board of Control, offered Bradman work as a stockbroker if he would relocate to Adelaide and captain South Australia (SA). Unknown to the public, the SA Cricket Association (SACA) instigated Hodgetts' approach and subsidised Bradman's wage.[65] Although his wife was hesitant about moving, Bradman eventually agreed to the deal in February 1934.[66]

Declining health and a brush with death

In his farewell season for NSW, Bradman averaged 132.44, his best yet.[27] He was appointed vice-captain for the 1934 tour of England. However, "he was unwell for much of the [English] summer, and reports in newspapers hinted that he was suffering from heart trouble".[67] Although he again started with a double century at Worcester, his famed concentration soon deserted him. *Wisden* wrote:[68]

... there were many occasions on which he was out to wild strokes. Indeed at one period he created the impression that, to some extent, he had lost control of himself and went in to bat with an almost complete disregard for anything in the shape of a defensive stroke.

Online image: Cigarette card distributed during the 1934 Ashes series

At one stage, Bradman went 13 first-class innings without a century, the longest such spell of his career,[69] prompting suggestions that Bodyline had eroded his confidence and altered his technique.[68] After three Tests, the series was one one and Bradman had scored 133 runs in five innings. The Australians travelled to Sheffield and played a warm up game before the Fourth Test. Bradman started slowly and then, "... the old Bradman [was] back with us, in the twinkling of an eye, almost".[70] He went on to make 140, with the last 90 runs coming in just 45 minutes. On the opening day of the Fourth Test at Headingley (Leeds), England were out for 200, but Australia slumped to 3/39, losing the third wicket from the last ball of the day.[71] Listed to bat at number five, Bradman would start his innings the next day.

That evening, Bradman declined an invitation to dinner from Neville Cardus, telling the journalist that he wanted an early night because the team needed him to make a double century the next day. Cardus pointed out that his previous innings on the ground was 334, and the law of averages was against another such score. Bradman told Cardus, "I don't believe in the law of averages".[72] In the event, Bradman batted all of the second day and into the third, putting on a world record partnership of 388 with Bill Ponsford.[73][74] When he was finally out for 304 (473 balls, 43 fours and 2 sixes), Australia had a lead of 350 runs, but rain prevented them from forcing a victory. The effort of the lengthy innings stretched Bradman's reserves of energy, and he did not play again until the Fifth Test at The Oval, the match that would decide the Ashes.[75]

In the first innings at The Oval, Bradman and Ponsford recorded an even more massive partnership, this time 451 runs. It had taken them less than a month to break the record they had set at Headingley; this new world record was to last 57 years.[73] Bradman's share of the stand was 244 from 271 balls, and the Australian total of 701 set up victory by 562 runs. For the fourth time in five series, the Ashes changed hands.[76] England would not recover them again until after Bradman's retirement.

Seemingly restored to full health, Bradman blazed two centuries in the last two games of the tour. However, when he returned to London to prepare for the trip home, he experienced severe abdominal pain. It took a doctor more than 24 hours to diagnose acute appendicitis and a surgeon operated immediately. Bradman lost a lot of blood during the four-hour procedure and peritonitis set in. Penicillin and sulphonamides were still experimental treatments at this time; peritonitis was usually a fatal condition.[77] On 25 September, the hospital issued a statement that Bradman was struggling for his life and that blood donors were needed urgently.[78]

"The effect of the announcement was little short of spectacular".[77] The hospital could not deal with the number of donors, and closed its switchboard in the face of the avalanche of telephone calls generated by the news. Journalists were asked by their editors to prepare obituaries. Teammate Bill O'Reilly took a call from King George's secretary asking that the King be kept informed of the situation.[78] Jessie Bradman started the month-long journey to London as soon as she received the news. En route, she heard a rumour that her husband had died.[77] A telephone call clarified the situation and by the time she reached London, Bradman had begun a slow recovery.

He followed medical advice to convalesce, taking several months to return to Australia and missing the 1934 35 Australian season.[15]

Internal politics and the Test captaincy

Online image: Bradman walking out to bat in the Third Test against England at the Melbourne Cricket Ground in 1937. His 270 runs won the match for Australia and has been rated the greatest innings of all time.

There was off-field intrigue in Australian cricket during the antipodean winter of 1935. Australia, scheduled to make a tour of South Africa at the end of the year, needed to replace the retired Bill Woodfull as captain. The Board of Control wanted Bradman to lead the team, yet, on 8 August, the Board announced Bradman's withdrawal from the team due to a lack of fitness. Surprisingly, in the light of this announcement, Bradman led the South Australian team in a full programme of matches that season.[79]

The captaincy was given to Vic Richardson, Bradman's predecessor as South Australian captain.[80] Cricket author Chris Harte's analysis of the situation is that a prior (unspecified) commercial agreement forced Bradman to remain in Australia.[81] Harte attributed an ulterior motive to his relocation: the off-field behaviour of Richardson and other South Australian players had displeased the South Australia Cricket Association (SACA), which was looking for new leadership. To help improve discipline, Bradman became a committeeman of the SACA, and a selector of the South Australian and Australian teams.[82] He took his adopted state to its first Sheffield Shield title for 10 years, Bradman weighing in with personal contributions of 233 against Queensland and 357 against Victoria. He finished the season with 369 (in 233 minutes), a South Australian record, made against the Tasmanian Tigers. The bowler who dismissed him, Reginald Townley, would later become leader of the Tasmanian Liberal Party.[79]

Australia defeated South Africa 4 0 and senior players such as Bill O'Reilly were pointed in their comments about the enjoyment of playing under Richardson's captaincy.[83] A group of players who were openly hostile toward Bradman formed during the tour. For some, the prospect of playing under Bradman was daunting, as was the knowledge that he would additionally be sitting in judgement of their abilities in his role as a selector.[84]

To start the new season, the Test side played a "Rest of Australia" team, captained by Bradman, at Sydney in early October 1936. The Test XI suffered a big defeat, due to Bradman's 212 and a haul of 12 wickets taken by leg-spinner Frank Ward.[85] Bradman let the members of the Test team know that despite their recent success, the team still required improvement.[84] Shortly afterwards, Bradman's first child was born on 28 October, but died the next day. He took time out of cricket for two weeks and on his return made 192 in three hours against Victoria in the last match before the beginning of the Ashes series.

The Test selectors made five changes to the team who had played in the previous Test match. Significantly, Australia's most successful bowler Clarrie Grimmett was replaced by Ward, one of four players making their debut. Bradman's role in Grimmett's omission from the team was controversial and it became a theme that dogged Bradman as Grimmett continued to be prolific in domestic cricket while his successors were ineffective he was regarded as having finished the veteran bowler's Test career in a political purge.[86]

Online image: Bradman and England captain Gubby Allen toss at the start of the 1936 37 Ashes series. The five Tests drew more than 950,000 spectators including a world record 350,534 to the Third Test at Melbourne.

Australia fell to successive defeats in the opening two Tests,[87] Bradman making two ducks in his four innings, and it seemed that the captaincy was affecting his form.[64] The selectors made another four changes to the team for the Third Test at Melbourne.

Bradman won the toss on New Year's Day 1937, but again failed with the bat, scoring just 13. The Australians could not take advantage of a pitch that favoured batting, and finished the day at 6/181. On the second day, rain dramatically altered the course of the game. With the sun drying the pitch (in those days, covers could not be used during matches) Bradman declared to get England in to bat while the pitch was "sticky"; England also declared to get Australia back in, conceding a lead of 124. Bradman countered by reversing his batting order to protect his run-makers while conditions improved. The ploy worked and Bradman went in at number seven. In an innings spread over three days, he battled influenza while scoring 270 off 375 balls, sharing a record partnership of 346 with Jack Fingleton,[88] and Australia went on to victory. In 2001, *Wisden* rated this performance as the best Test match innings of all time.[89]

The next Test, at the Adelaide Oval, was fairly even until Bradman played another patient second innings, making 212 from 395 balls. Australia levelled the series when the erratic[90] left-arm spinner "Chuck" Fleetwood-Smith bowled Australia to victory. In the series-deciding Fifth Test, Bradman returned to a more aggressive style in top-scoring with 169 (off 191 balls) in Australia's 604 and Australia won by an innings.[91] Australia's achievement of winning a series after losing the first two Tests has, of 2009, not been equalled in Test cricket.[92]

End of an era

During the 1938 tour of England, Bradman played the most consistent cricket of his career.[93] He needed to score heavily as England had a strengthened batting line-up, while the Australian bowling was over-reliant on O'Reilly.[93] Grimmett was overlooked, but Jack Fingleton made the team, so the clique of anti-Bradman players remained.[6] Playing 26 innings on tour, Bradman recorded 13 centuries (a new Australian record) and again made 1,000 first-class runs before the end of May, becoming the only player to do so twice.[94] In scoring 2,429 runs, Bradman achieved the highest average ever recorded in an English season: 115.66.[93]

Online image: Bradman (left, with his vice-captain Stan McCabe) walks out to bat at Perth, during a preliminary match to the 1938 tour of England. Bradman scored 102.

In the First Test, England amassed a big first innings score and looked likely to win, but Stan McCabe made 232 for Australia, a performance Bradman rated as the best he had ever seen. With Australia forced to follow-on, Bradman fought hard to ensure McCabe's effort was not in vain, and he secured the draw with 144 not out.[95] It was the slowest Test hundred of his career and he played a similar innings of 102 not out in the next Test as Australia struggled to another draw.[96] Rain completely washed out the Third Test at Manchester.[97]

Australia's opportunity came at Headingley, a Test described by Bradman as the best he ever played in.[98] England batted first and made 223. During the Australian innings, Bradman backed himself by opting to bat on in poor light conditions, when he had the option to go off.[99] He scored 103 out of a total of 242 and the gamble paid off, as it meant there was sufficient time to push for victory when an England collapse left them a target of only 107 to win. Australia slumped to 4/61, with Bradman out for 16. An approaching storm threatened to wash the game out, but the poor weather held off and Australia managed to secure the win, a victory that retained the Ashes.[99] For the only time in his life, the tension of the occasion got to Bradman and he could not watch the closing stages of play, a reflection of the pressure that he felt all tour: he described the captaincy as "exhausting" and said he "found it difficult to keep going".[98]

Online image: "Australia's greatest batsman". Caricature by ex-Australian Test player Arthur Mailey (c. 1939).

The euphoria of securing the Ashes preceded Australia's heaviest defeat. At The Oval, England amassed a world record of 7/903 and their opening batsman Len Hutton scored an individual world record, by making 364.[100][101] In an attempt to relieve the burden on his bowlers, Bradman took a rare turn at bowling. During his third over, he fractured his ankle and teammates carried him from the ground.[100] With Bradman injured and Fingleton unable to bat because of a leg muscle strain,[100][102] Australia were thrashed by an innings and 579 runs, which remains the largest margin in Test cricket history.[103] Unfit to complete the tour, Bradman left the team in the hands of vice-captain Stan McCabe. At this point, Bradman felt that the burden of captaincy would prevent him from touring England again, although he did not make his doubts public.[98]

Despite the pressure of captaincy, Bradman's batting form remained supreme. An experienced, mature player now commonly called "The Don" had replaced the blitzing style of his early days as the "Boy from Bowral".[104] In 1938 39, he led SA to the

Sheffield Shield and made a century in six consecutive innings to equal the world record of CB Fry.[105] Bradman totalled 21 first-class centuries in 34 innings, from the beginning of the 1938 tour of England (including preliminary games in Australia) until early 1939.

The next season, Bradman made an abortive bid to join the Victoria State side. The Melbourne Cricket Club advertised the position of club secretary and he was led to believe that if he applied, he would get the job.[106] The position, which had been held by Hugh Trumble until his death in August 1938, was one of the most prestigious jobs in Australian cricket. The annual salary of $1,000 would make Bradman financially secure while allowing him to retain a connection with the game.[107] On 18 January 1939, the club's committee, on the casting vote of the chairman, chose ex-Test batsman Vernon Ransford over Bradman.[107][108]

The 1939 40 season was Bradman's most productive ever for SA: 1,448 runs at an average of 144.8.[27] He made three double centuries, including 251 not out against NSW, the innings that he rated the best he ever played in the Sheffield Shield, as he tamed Bill O'Reilly at the height of his form.[109] However, it was the end of an era. The outbreak of World War Two led to the indefinite postponement of all cricket tours, and the suspension of the Sheffield Shield competition.[110]

Troubled war years

Online image: Bradman's high backlift and lengthy forward stride were characteristic.

Bradman joined the Royal Australian Air Force (RAAF) on 28 June 1940 and was passed fit for air crew duty.[111] The RAAF had more recruits than it could equip and train and Bradman spent four months in Adelaide before the Governor-General of Australia, Lord Gowrie, persuaded Bradman to transfer to the army, a move that was criticised as a safer option for him.[6] Given the rank of Lieutenant, he was posted to the Army School of Physical Training at Frankston, Victoria, to act as a divisional supervisor of physical training. The exertion of the job aggravated his chronic muscular problems, diagnosed as fibrositis. Surprisingly, in light of his batting prowess, a routine army test revealed that Bradman had poor eyesight.[112]

Invalided out of service in June 1941, Bradman spent months recuperating, unable even to shave himself or comb his hair due to the extent of the muscular pain he suffered. He resumed stockbroking during 1942. In his biography of Bradman, Charles Williams expounded the theory that the physical problems were psychosomatic, induced by stress and possibly depression; Bradman read the book's manuscript and did not disagree.[113] Had any cricket been played at this time, he would not have been available. Although he found some relief in 1945 when referred to the Melbourne masseur Ern Saunders, Bradman permanently lost the feeling in the thumb and index finger of his (dominant) right hand.[114]

In June 1945, Bradman faced a financial crisis when the firm of Harry Hodgetts collapsed due to fraud and embezzlement.[115] Bradman moved quickly to set up his own business, utilizing Hodgetts' client list and his old office in Grenfell Street, Adelaide. The fallout led to a prison term for Hodgetts, and left a stigma attached to Bradman's name in the city's business community for many years.[116]

However, the SA Cricket Association had no hesitation in appointing Bradman as their delegate to the Board of Control in place of Hodgetts. Now working alongside some of the men he had battled in the 1930s, Bradman quickly became a leading light in the administration of the game. With the resumption of international cricket, he was once more appointed a Test selector, and played a major role in planning for post-war cricket.[117]

"The ghost of a once great cricketer"

Online image: Bradman and Barnes leave the field for an adjournment as both head towards 234.

In 1945 46, Bradman suffered regular bouts of fibrositis while coming to terms with increased administrative duties and the establishment of his business.[118] He played for SA in two matches to help with the re-establishment of first-class cricket and later described his batting as "painstaking".[119] Batting against the Australian Services cricket team, Bradman scored 112 in less than two hours, yet Dick Whitington (playing for the Services) wrote, "I have seen today the ghost of a once great cricketer".[120] Bradman declined a tour of New Zealand and spent the winter of 1946 wondering whether he had played his last match. With the English team due to arrive for the Ashes series, the media and the public were anxious to know if Bradman would lead Australia.[121] His doctor recommended against a return to the game.[122] Encouraged by his wife, Bradman agreed to play in lead-up fixtures to the Test series.[123] After hitting two centuries, Bradman made himself available for the First Test at The Gabba.

Controversy emerged as early as the first day of the series. After compiling an uneasy 28 runs, Bradman hit a ball to the gully fieldsman, Jack Ikin. An appeal for a catch was denied in the umpire's contentious ruling that it was a bump ball.[124] At the end of the over, England captain Wally Hammond spoke with Bradman and criticised him for not "walking"; "from then on the series was a cricketing war just when most people desired peace", Whitington wrote.[125] Bradman regained his finest pre-war form in making 187, followed by 234 during the Second Test at Sydney. Australia won both matches by an innings. Jack Fingleton speculated that had the decision at Brisbane gone against him, Bradman would have retired, such were his fitness problems.[126] In the remainder of the series, Bradman made three half-centuries in six innings, but was unable to make another century; nevertheless, his team won handsomely, 3 0. He was the leading batsman on either side, with an average of 97.14. Nearly 850,000 spectators watched the Tests, which helped lift public spirits after the war.[127]

Century of centuries and "The Invincibles"

Main article: Donald Bradman with the Australian cricket team in England in 1948

See also: Australian cricket team in England in 1948 and 1948 Ashes series

Online image: The 1948 "Invincibles" *en route* to England. Bradman is standing with hat in hand, third from the left.

India made its first tour of Australia in the 1947 48 season. On 15 November, Bradman made 172 against them for an Australian XI at Sydney, his 100th first-class century.[128] The first non-Englishman to achieve the milestone, Bradman remains the only Australian to have done so.[129] In five Tests, he scored 715 runs (at 178.75 average). His last double century (201) came at Adelaide, and he scored a century in each innings of the Melbourne Test.[130] On the eve of the Fifth Test, he announced that the match would be his last in Australia, although he would tour England as a farewell.[131]

Australia had assembled one of the great teams of cricket history.[132] Bradman made it known that he wanted to go through the tour unbeaten,[50] a feat never accomplished, before or since.[133] English spectators were drawn to the matches knowing that it would be their last opportunity to see Bradman in action. RC Robertson-Glasgow observed of Bradman that:[27]

Next to Mr. Winston Churchill, he was the most celebrated man in England during the summer of 1948. His appearances throughout the country were like one continuous farewell matinée. At last his batting showed human fallibility. Often, especially at the start of the innings, he played where the ball wasn't, and spectators rubbed their eyes.

Despite his waning powers, Bradman compiled 11 centuries on the tour, amassing 2,428 runs (average 89.92).[27] His highest score of the tour (187) came against Essex, when Australia compiled a world record of 721 runs in a day. In the Tests, he scored a century at Nottingham, but the performance most like his pre-war exploits came in the Fourth Test at Leeds. England declared on the last morning of the game, setting Australia a world record 404 runs to win in only 345 minutes on a heavily worn wicket. In partnership with Arthur Morris (182), Bradman reeled off 173 not out and the match was won with 15 minutes to spare. The journalist Ray Robinson called the victory "the 'finest ever' in its conquest of seemingly insuperable odds".[134]

In the final Test at The Oval, Bradman walked out to bat in Australia's first innings. He received a standing ovation from the crowd and three cheers from the opposition. His Test batting average stood at 101.39. Facing the wrist-spin of Eric Hollies, Bradman pushed forward to the second ball that he faced, was deceived by a googly, and bowled between bat and pad for a duck. An England batting collapse resulted in an innings defeat, denying Bradman the opportunity to bat again and so his career average finished at 99.94; if he had scored just four runs in his last innings, it would have been 100. A story developed over the years that claimed Bradman missed the ball because of tears in his eyes, a claim Bradman denied for the rest of his life.[64]

The Australian team won the Ashes 4 0, completed the tour unbeaten, and have entered history as "The Invincibles".[135] Just as Bradman's legend grew, rather than diminished, over the years, so too has the reputation of the 1948 team. For Bradman, it was the most personally fulfilling period of his playing days, as the divisiveness of the 1930s had passed. He wrote:[136]

Knowing the personnel, I was confident that here at last was the great opportunity which I had longed for. A team of cricketers whose respect and loyalty were unquestioned, who would regard me in a fatherly sense and listen to my advice, follow my guidance and not question my handling of affairs ... there are no longer any fears that they will query the wisdom of what you do. The result is a sense of freedom to give full reign to your own creative ability and personal judgment.

With Bradman now retired from professional cricket, RC Robertson-Glasgow wrote of the English reaction "... a miracle has been removed from among us. So must ancient Italy have felt when she heard of the death of Hannibal".[27]

After cricket

After his return to Australia, Bradman played in his own Testimonial match at Melbourne, scoring his 117th and last century, and receiving $9,342 in proceeds.[137] In the 1949 New Year's Honours List, he was made a Knight Bachelor[138] for his services to the game, being the only Australian cricketer ever to be knighted.[139] The following year he published a memoir, *Farewell to Cricket*.[140] Bradman accepted offers from the *Daily Mail* to travel with, and write about, the 1953 and 1956 Australian teams in England. *The Art of Cricket*, his final book published in 1958, is an instructional manual.[6]

Bradman retired from his stockbroking business in June 1954, depending on the "comfortable" income earned as a board member of 16 publicly listed companies.[141] His highest profile affiliation was with Argo Investments Limited, where he was chairman for a number of years. Charles Williams commented that, "[b]usiness was excluded on medical grounds, [so] the only sensible alternative was a career in the administration of the game which he loved and to which he had given most of his active life".[142]

Bradman was honoured at a number of cricket grounds, notably when his portrait was hung in the Long Room at Lord's; until Shane Warne's portrait was added in 2005, Bradman was one of just three Australians to be honoured in this way.[143][144][145] Bradman inaugurated a "Bradman Stand" at the Sydney Cricket Ground in January 1974;[146] the Adelaide Oval also opened a Bradman Stand in 1990.[147] Later in

1974, he attended a Lord's Taverners function in London where he experienced heart problems,[148] which forced him to limit his public appearances to select occasions only. With his wife, Bradman returned to Bowral in 1976, where the new cricket ground was named in his honour.[149] He gave the keynote speech at the historic Centenary Test at Melbourne in 1977.[150]

On 16 June 1979, the Australian government awarded Bradman the nation's second-highest civilian honour at that time, Companion of the Order of Australia (AC), "in recognition of service to the sport of cricket and cricket administration".[151] In 1980, he resigned from the ACB, to lead a more secluded life.

Administrative career

See also: Controversies involving Donald Bradman

In addition to acting as one of South Australia's delegates to the Board of Control from 1945 to 1980, Bradman was a committee member of the SACA between 1935 and 1986. It is estimated that he attended 1,713 SACA meetings during this half century of service. Aside from two years in the early 1950s, he filled a selector's berth for the Test team between 1936 and 1971.[152]

Cricket saw an increase in defensive play during the 1950s. As a selector, Bradman favoured attacking, positive cricketers who entertained the paying public. He formed an alliance with Australian captain Richie Benaud, seeking more attractive play,[153] with some success.[154] He served two high-profile periods as Chairman of the Board of Control, in 1960 63 and 1969 72.[155] During the first, he dealt with the growing prevalence of illegal bowling actions in the game, a problem that he adjudged "the most complex I have known in cricket, because it is not a matter of fact but of opinion".[6] The major controversy of his second stint was a proposed tour of Australia by South Africa in 1971 72. On Bradman's recommendation, the series was cancelled.[156]

Bradman was more than a cricket player nonpareil. He was ... an astute and progressive administrator; an expansive thinker, philosopher and writer on the game. Indeed, in some respects, he was as powerful, persuasive and influential a figure off the ground as he was on it.

Mike Coward[157]

In the late 1970s, Bradman played an important role during the World Series Cricket schism as a member of a special Australian Cricket Board committee formed to handle the crisis. He was criticised for not airing an opinion, but he dealt with World Series Cricket far more pragmatically than other administrators.[158] Richie Benaud described Bradman as "a brilliant administrator and businessman", warning that he was not to be underestimated.[159] As Australian captain, Ian Chappell fought with

Bradman over the issue of player remuneration in the early 1970s and has suggested that Bradman was parsimonious:[160]

I ... thought to myself, 'Ian, did you just ask Bradman to fill your wallet with money?' Bradman's harangue confirmed my suspicions that the players were going to have a hard time extracting more money from the ACB.

Later years and legacy

Cricket writer David Frith summed up the paradox of the continuing fascination with Bradman:[161]

As the years passed, with no lessening of his reclusiveness, so his public stature continued to grow, until the sense of reverence and unquestioning worship left many of his contemporaries scratching their heads in wondering admiration.

On 10 December 1985, Bradman was the first of 120 inaugural inductees into the Sport Australia Hall of Fame.[162] He spoke of his philosophy for considering the stature of athletes:[1]

When considering the stature of an athlete or for that matter any person, I set great store in certain qualities which I believe to be essential in addition to skill. They are that the person conducts his of her life with dignity, with integrity, courage, and perhaps most of all, with modesty. These virtues are totally compatible with pride, ambition, and competitiveness.

Although modest about his own abilities and generous in his praise of other cricketers, Bradman was fully aware of the talents he possessed as a player;[163] there is some evidence that he sought to influence his legacy.[164] During the 1980s and 1990s, Bradman carefully selected the people to whom he gave interviews,[164] assisting Michael Page, Roland Perry and Charles Williams, who all produced biographical works about him. Bradman also agreed to an extensive interview for ABC radio, broadcast as *Bradman: The Don Declares* in eight 55-minute episodes during 1988.[165]

Online image: The Bradman Stand (named in 1990) at the Adelaide Oval

The most significant of these legacy projects was a museum, opened in 1987 at the Bradman Oval in Bowral.[166] This organisation was reformed in 1993 as a non-profit charitable Trust, called the Bradman Foundation.[167] When the Australian Cricket Hall of Fame was created in 1996, Bradman was made one of its 10 inaugural members.[168] In 2000, Bradman was selected by cricket experts as one of five *Wisden Cricketers of the Century*. Each of the 100 members of the panel were able to select five cricketers: all 100 voted for Bradman.[169]

After his wife's death in 1997, Bradman suffered "a discernible and not unexpected wilting of spirit".[170] The next year, on his 90th birthday, he hosted a meeting with his two favourite modern players, Shane Warne and Sachin Tendulkar,[171] but he was not seen in his familiar place at the Adelaide Oval again.[172] Hospitalised with pneumonia in December 2000, he returned home in the New Year and died there on 25 February 2001, aged 92.[173]

A memorial service to mark Bradman's life was held on 25 March 2001 at St Peter's Anglican Cathedral, Adelaide. The service was attended by a host of former and current Test cricketers, as well as Australia's then prime minister, John Howard, leader of the opposition Kim Beazley and former prime minister Bob Hawke. Eulogies were given by Richie Benaud and Governor-General Sir William Deane. The service was broadcast live on ABC Television to a viewing audience of 1.45 million.[174]

Bradman's life and achievements were recognised in Australia with two notable issues. Three years before he died, he became the first living Australian to be featured on an Australian postage stamp.[175] After his death, the Australian Government produced a 20 cent coin to commemorate his life.[176]

Family life

Online image: A collection of Bradman's private letters was published in 2004, giving researchers new insights into Bradman's personal life.

Bradman first met Jessie Martha Menzies in 1920 when she boarded with the Bradman family, to be closer to school in Bowral. The couple married at St Paul's Anglican Church at Burwood, Sydney on 30 April 1932.[15] During their 65-year marriage, Jessie was "shrewd, reliable, selfless, and above all, uncomplicated ... she was the perfect foil to his concentrated, and occasionally mercurial character".[177] Bradman paid tribute to his wife numerous times, once saying succinctly, "I would never have achieved what I achieved without Jessie".[178]

The Bradmans lived in the same modest, suburban house in Holden Street, Kensington Park in Adelaide for all but the first three years of their married life.[179] They experienced much personal tragedy in raising their children. Their first-born son died as an infant in 1936,[180] their second son, John (born in 1939) contracted polio,[181] and their daughter, Shirley, born in 1941, had cerebral palsy since her birth.[182] His family name proved a burden for John Bradman; he changed his last name to Bradsen by deed poll in 1972. Although claims were made that he became estranged from his father, it was more a matter of "the pair inhabit[ing] different worlds".[183] After the cricketer's death, a collection of personal letters written by Bradman to his close friend Rohan Rivett between 1953 and 1977 was released and gave researchers new insights into Bradman's family life, including the strain between father and son.[184]

Bradman's reclusiveness in later life is partly attributable to the on-going health problems of his wife, particularly following the open-heart surgery Jessie underwent in her 60s.[148] Lady Bradman died in 1997, aged 88, from cancer.[185] This had a dispiriting effect on Bradman, but the relationship with his son improved, to the extent that John resolved to change his name back to Bradman.[186] Since his father's death, John Bradman has become the spokesperson for the family and has been involved in defending the Bradman legacy in a number of disputes.[187][188] The relationship between Bradman and his wider family is less clear, although nine months after Bradman's death, his nephew Paul Bradman criticised him as a "snob" and a "loner" who forgot his connections in Bowral and who failed to attend the funerals of Paul's mother and father.[189]

Style

Main article: Donald Bradman's batting technique

Online image: Bradman hooks English left-arm fast bowler Bill Voce during the 1936 37 series. The position of Bradman's left foot in relation to the stumps is an example of how he used the crease when batting.

Bradman's early development was shaped by the high bounce of the ball on matting-over-concrete pitches. He favoured "horizontal-bat" shots (such as the hook, pull and cut) to deal with the bounce and devised a unique grip on the bat handle that would accommodate these strokes without compromising his ability to defend. Employing a side-on stance at the wicket, Bradman kept perfectly still as the bowler ran in.[190] His backswing had a "crooked" look that troubled his early critics, but he resisted entreaties to change.[191] His backswing kept his hands in close to the body, leaving him perfectly balanced and able to change his stroke mid-swing, if need be.[192] Another telling factor was the decisiveness of Bradman's footwork. He "used the crease" by either coming metres down the wicket to drive, or playing so far back that his feet ended up level with the stumps when playing the cut, hook or pull.[193]

Bradman's game evolved with experience. He temporarily adapted his technique during the Bodyline series, deliberately moving around the crease in an attempt to score from the short-pitched deliveries.[194] At his peak, in the mid-1930s, he had the ability to switch between a defensive and attacking approach as the occasion demanded. After the Second World War, he adjusted to bat within the limitations set by his age, becoming a steady "accumulator" of runs.[195] However, Bradman never truly mastered batting on sticky wickets. *Wisden* commented, "[i]f there really is a blemish on his amazing record it is ... the absence of a significant innings on one of those 'sticky dogs' of old".[1]

In popular culture

Main article: Donald Bradman in popular culture

Online image: Bradman statue outside the Adelaide Oval

Bradman's name has become an archetypal name for outstanding excellence, both within cricket and in the wider world. The term **Bradmanesque** has been coined and is used both within and without cricketing circles.[196] Steve Waugh described Sri Lankan Muttiah Muralitharan as the "the Don Bradman of bowling",[197] while former Australian Prime Minister John Howard was called "the Don Bradman of politics" by his Liberal Party colleague Joe Hockey.[198]

Bradman has been the subject of more biographies than any other Australian, apart from the outlaw Ned Kelly.[199] Bradman himself wrote four books: *Don Bradman's Book The Story of My Cricketing Life with Hints on Batting, Bowling and Fielding* (1930), *My Cricketing Life* (1938), *Farewell to Cricket* (1950) and *The Art of Cricket* (1958). The story of the Bodyline series was retold in a 1984 television mini-series.[200]

Bradman is immortalised in three popular songs from different eras, "Our Don Bradman" (1930s, by Jack O'Hagan),[201] "Bradman" (1980s, by Paul Kelly),[202] and "Sir Don", (a tribute by John Williamson performed at Bradman's memorial service).[203] Bradman recorded several songs accompanying himself and others on piano in the early 1930s, including "Every Day Is A Rainbow Day For Me".[204] In 2000, the Australian Government made it illegal for the names of corporations to suggest a link to "Sir Donald Bradman", if such a link does not in fact exist.[205] Other entities with similar protection are the Australian and foreign governments, the British Royal Family and the Returned and Services League of Australia.[206]

Statistical summary

Test match performance

Online image: A graph of Bradman's Test career batting performances. The red bars indicate his innings, and the blue line the average of his 10 most recent innings. The blue dots indicate innings in which Bradman finished not out.

: Batting[207]: Bowling[208]

- o Opposition: Matches: Runs: Average: High Score: 100 / 50: Runs: Wickets: Average: Best (Inns)
- o England: 37: 5028: 89.78: 334: 19/12: 51: 1: 51.00: 1/23
- o India: 5: 715: 178.75: 201: 4/1: 4: 0: :
- o South Africa: 5: 806: 201.50: 299*: 4/0: 2: 0: :
- o West Indies: 5: 447: 74.50: 223: 2/0: 15: 1: 15.00: 1/8
- o Overall: 52: 6996: 99.94: 334: 29/13: 72: 2: 36.00: 1/8

First-class performance

: Innings: Not Out: Highest: Aggregate: Average: 100s: 100s/inns

- Ashes Tests: 63: 7: 334: 5,028: 89.78: 19: 30.2%
- All Tests: 80: 10: 334: 6,996: 99.94: 29: 36.3%
- Sheffield Shield: 96: 15: 452*: 8,926: 110.19: 36: 37.5%
- All First Class: 338: 43: 452*: 28,067: 95.10: 117: 34.6%
- Grade: 93: 17: 303: 6,598: 86.80: 28: 30.1%
- All Second Class: 331: 64: 320*: 22,664: 84.80: 94: 28.4%
- **Grand Total: 669: 107: 452*: 50,731: 90.27: 211: 31.5%**
- Statistics from Bradman Museum.[209]

Test records

See also: List of international cricket centuries by Donald Bradman

Bradman still holds the following significant records for Test match cricket:

- Highest career batting average (minimum 20 innings): 99.94[210]
- Highest series batting average (5 Test series): 201.50 (1931 32)[211]
- Highest ratio of centuries per innings played: 36.25% (29 centuries from 80 innings)[212]
- Highest 5th wicket partnership: 405 (with Sid Barnes, 1946 47)[213]
- Highest 6th wicket partnership: 346 (with Jack Fingleton, 1936 37)[214]
- Highest score by a number 5 batsman: 304 (1934)[215]
- Highest score by a number 7 batsman: 270 (1936 37)[215]
- Most runs against one opponent: 5,028 (v England)[216]
- Most runs in one series: 974 (1930)[217]
- Most centuries scored in a single session of play: 6 (1 pre lunch, 2 lunch-tea, 3 tea-stumps)[218]
- Most runs in one day's play: 309 (1930)[219]
- Most double centuries: 12[220]
- Most double centuries in a series: 3 (1930)[221]
- Most triple centuries: 2 (equal with Brian Lara and Virender Sehwag)[222]
- Most consecutive matches in which he made a century: 6 (the last three Tests in 1936 37, and the first three Tests in 1938)[223]
- Bradman has averaged over 100 in seven different calendar years (*qualification 400 runs). No other player has achieved this in more than two calendar years.
- Fastest player to reach 2000 (in 22 innings),[224] 3000 (33 innings),[225] 4000 (48 innings),[226] 5000 (56 innings)[227] and 6000 (68 innings)[228] Test runs.

Cricket context

Donald Bradman (AUS): 99.94

- Graeme Pollock (SAF): 60.97
- George Headley (WI): 60.83
- Herbert Sutcliffe (ENG): 60.73
- Eddie Paynter (ENG): 59.23
- Ken Barrington (ENG): 58.67

o Everton Weekes (WI): 58.61
o Wally Hammond (ENG): 58.45
o Garfield Sobers (WI): 57.78
o Jack Hobbs (ENG): 56.94
o Clyde Walcott (WI): 56.68
o Len Hutton (ENG): 56.67
o Ernest Tyldesley (ENG): 55.00
o Charlie Davis (WI): 54.20
o Vinod Kambli (IND): 54.20
o *Source: Cricinfo Qualification:* **20** *completed innings, career completed.*

Bradman's Test batting average of 99.94 has become one of cricket's most famous, iconic statistics.[34] No other player who has played more than 20 Test match innings has finished with a Test average of more than 61.[210] Bradman scored centuries at a rate better than one every three innings in 80 Test innings, Bradman scored 29 centuries.[229] Only seven players have surpassed his total, all at a much slower rate: Sachin Tendulkar (who required 159 innings to do so), Matthew Hayden (167 innings), Ricky Ponting (170 innings), Sunil Gavaskar (174 innings), Jacques Kallis (200 innings), Brian Lara (205 innings) and Steve Waugh (247 innings).[229] He converted 41.4% of his centuries into double centuries.[230] His total of 12 Test double hundreds (in 15% of his innings) is the most achieved by any batsman.[220] Next best is Brian Lara with 9 in 232 innings (4%), Walter Hammond with 7 in 140 innings (5%) and Kumar Sangakkara 6 in 110 innings (5%).[220]

World sport context

Wisden hailed Bradman as, "the greatest phenomenon in the history of cricket, indeed in the history of all ball games".[1] Statistician Charles Davis analysed the statistics for several prominent sportsmen by comparing the number of standard deviations that they stand above the mean for their sport.[231] The top performers in his selected sports are:[232]

Athlete: Sport: Statistic: Standard deviations

o Bradman: Cricket: Batting average: 4.4
o Pelé: Association football: Goals per game: 3.7
o Ty Cobb: Baseball: Batting average: 3.6
o Jack Nicklaus: Golf: Major titles: 3.5
o Michael Jordan: Basketball: Points per game: 3.4

The statistics show that "no other athlete dominates an international sport to the extent that Bradman does cricket".[2] In order to post a similarly dominant career statistic as Bradman, a baseball batter would need a career batting average of .392, while a basketball player would need to score an average of 43.0 points per game.[232] The respective records are .366 and 30.1.[232]

When Bradman died, *Time* magazine allocated a space in its "Milestones" column for an obituary:[233]

... Australian icon considered by many to be the pre-eminent sportsman of all time ... One of Australia's most beloved heroes, he was revered abroad as well. When Nelson Mandela was released after 27 years in prison, his first question to an Australian visitor was, "Is Sir Donald Bradman still alive?"

Honoured by Wisden

In the 1963 edition of *Wisden Cricketers' Almanack*, Bradman was selected by Neville Cardus as one the Six Giants of the Wisden Century. This was a special commemorative selection requested by Wisden for its 100th edition.[234] The other five players chosen were:

- Sydney Barnes
- W G Grace
- Jack Hobbs
- Tom Richardson
- Victor Trumper

Notes

- 1. "Sir Donald Bradman player profile". *Cricinfo*. Retrieved 2008-05-18. "Sir Donald Bradman of Australia was, beyond any argument, the greatest batsman who ever lived and the greatest cricketer of the 20th century. Only WG Grace, in the formative years of the game, even remotely matched his status as a player."
- 2. Hutchins, Brett (2002). *Don Bradman: Challenging the Myth*. Cambridge University Press. pp. 21. ISBN 0521823846.
- 3. "Legislative Assembly of ACT". *Hansard*. 2001-02-28. Retrieved 2008-08-23.
- 4. "The Sports Factor (transcript)". *ABC Radio*. 2001-03-02. Retrieved 2008-08-23.
- 5. McGilvray (1986), pp 20 23.
- 6. Swanton, E. W. (2002 edition). ""A Personal Recollection"". *Wisden*. Retrieved 2007-08-03.
- 7. Haigh, Gideon (2002 edition). ""Beyond the Legend"". *Wisden*. Retrieved 2007-08-22.
- 8. The Don celebrated on commemorative $5 coin
- 9. "Sir Don Bradman inducted into the ICC Cricket Hall of Fame".
- 10. "Donald George Bradman". *Bradman Museum*. Retrieved 2008-08-23.
- 11. A stump is considerably narrower than a bat; the diameter of a golf ball is similarly smaller than that of a cricket ball.
- 12. "The Boy in Bowral (1911 1924)". *Bradman Foundation*. Retrieved 2008-06-27.
- 13. "Bradman Foundation: Biography.". Archived from the original on 2008-02-06. Bradman Museum. Retrieved on 21 August 2007.
- 14. Perry (1995), p 24.
- 15. Page, Michael (1984). "Bradman Digital Library: Essay by Michael Page". *Pan Macmillan Australia Pty Ltd*. Retrieved 2008-05-23.

- 16. Page (1983), pp 21 23.
- 17. Harte (1993), pp 300 302.
- 18. "St George District Cricket Club" (PDF). *St George District Cricket Club Inc.* Retrieved 2008-05-23.
- 19. Robinson (1981), p 138.
- 20. Bradman (1950), p 25.
- 21. "FAQs". *Bradman Museum.* Archived from the original on 2007-09-01. Retrieved 2008-08-23.
- 22. "1st Test Australia v England, match report". *Wisden.* 1930 edition. Retrieved 2007-08-07.
- 23. Whitington (1974), p 142.
- 24. Whitington (1974), p 147. This record was broken in the next Test when Australia's Archie Jackson hit 164 on debut at Adelaide.
- 25. "4th Test Australia v England, match report". *Wisden.* 1930 edition. Retrieved 2007-08-21.
- 26. Bradman (1950). See appendix.
- 27. Robertson-Glasgow, R. C. (1949 edition). ""A Miracle Has Been Removed From Among Us"". *Wisden.* Retrieved 2007-08-20.
- 28. Bradman (1950), p 29.
- 29. Quoted in Haigh 2008.
- 30. Quoted by Page (1983), p 49.
- 31. "Notes by the Editor". *Wisden.* 1931 edition. Retrieved 2008-05-14.
- 32. "Forgotten genius". *The Times.* London. Retrieved 2008-08-23.
- 33. Page (1983), p 361.
- 34. Haigh, Gideon. "Bradman's best: Speed without haste, risk without recklessness". *Inside Edge.* Retrieved 2008-05-23.
- 35. "Second Test match: England v Australia 1930". *Wisden.* 1931 edition. Retrieved 2008-05-23.
- 36. "Hundred before lunch". *Cricinfo.* Retrieved 2008-08-23.
- 37. "Most runs in a day". *Cricinfo.* Retrieved 2007-08-07.
- 38. Lynch, Steven (2004-04-12). "The progression of the record The highest score in Test cricket". *Cricinfo.* Retrieved 2008-08-23.
- 39. Eason (2004), p 336. Whitelaw gave each of the other Australian players an ashtray.
- 40. "Fifth Test Match: England v Australia 1930". *Wisden.* 1931 edition. Retrieved 2008-05-23.
- 41. Steen, Rob (2005-06-04). "The coming of 'Our Don'". *The Age.* Retrieved 2008-08-23.
- 42. "Sir Donald Bradman (1908 2001)". *BBC Sport.* Retrieved 2008-05-23.
- 43. "Test Matches Most runs in a series". *Cricinfo.* Retrieved 2008-04-24.
- 44. "Timeline". *The Bradman Foundation.* 2006. Retrieved 2008-05-28.
- 45. Harte (1993), p 327.
- 46. Cashman et al. (1996), p 573.
- 47. "South African team in Australia and New Zealand 1931 32". *Wisden.* 1933 edition. Retrieved 2008-05-23.
- 48. "Test matches: Most runs in an innings". *Cricinfo.* Retrieved 2008-05-23. The record was beaten by Bob Cowper, who scored 307 in 1965 66.
- 49. "DG Bradman Test matches Batting analysis". *Cricinfo.* Retrieved 2008-04-27.
- 50. "Sir Donald Bradman". *The Daily Telegraph.* 2001-11-22. Retrieved 2008-08-23.
- 51. Williams (1996), pp 78 81.

- o 52. "When the Don met the Babe". *Cricinfo*. Retrieved 2008-08-23.
- o 53. Quoted by Harte (1993), p 327. The rules of English billiards were changed to limit the prodigious breaks of Australian Walter Lindrum.
- o 54. Frith (2002), pp 40 41.
- o 55. Williams (1996), pp 90 91.
- o 56. Bradman (1950), p 60.
- o 57. Williamson, Martin. "Bodyline quotes". *Cricinfo*. Retrieved 2008-04-25.
- o 58. Whitington (1974), p 170.
- o 59. Williams (1996), pp 97 98.
- o 60. "2nd Test Australia v England, match report". *Wisden*. 1934 edition. Retrieved 2007-08-21.
- o 61. Roebuck, Peter (2004-02-11). "Bodyline consumed two nations". *The Age*. Retrieved 2008-08-23.
- o 62. Williams (1996), p 99.
- o 63. Fingleton (1949), p 198.
- o 64. "The Bradman interview (transcript)". *Cricinfo*. Retrieved 2007-08-22.
- o 65. Harte (1993), pp 352 353.
- o 66. Williams (1996), p 119 120.
- o 67. "Call back the medics". *Cricinfo*. Retrieved 2008-08-23.
- o 68. Southerton, S. J. (1935 edition). "The Australian team in England, 1934". *Wisden*. Retrieved 2008-04-25.
- o 69. "Player Oracle Reveals Results, DG Bradman". *Cricket Archive*. Retrieved 2008-05-19.
- o 70. Williams (1996), p 131.
- o 71. "Ponsford, Bradman and the spin triplets". *Cricinfo*. Retrieved 2008-08-23.
- o 72. Rosenwater (1978), p 229.
- o 73. "Test matches Highest partnerships for any wicket". *Cricinfo*. Retrieved 2008-05-13.
- o 74. The previous mark had been 323, set in 1912.
- o 75. "4th Test England v Australia, match report". *Wisden*. 1935 edition. Retrieved 2007-08-21.
- o 76. "5th Test England v Australia, match report". *Wisden*. 1935 edition. Retrieved 2007-08-21.
- o 77. Williams (1996), pp 136 37.
- o 78. O'Reilly (1985), p 139.
- o 79. Bradman (1950), pp 94 97.
- o 80. "Vic Richardson player profile". *Cricinfo*. Retrieved 2008-06-17. Richardson's record in 14 Tests was 622 runs at 24.88. Against South Africa, he made 84 runs in 5 innings.
- o 81. Harte (1993), p 360.
- o 82. Harte (1993), p 352.
- o 83. O'Reilly (1985), pp 144 145.
- o 84. Williams (1996), p 148.
- o 85. Harte (1993), p 369.
- o 86. "Clarrie Grimmett player profile". *Cricinfo*. Retrieved 2008-08-23.
- o 87. "2nd Test Scorecard, 18 22 Dec 1936". *Cricinfo*. Retrieved 2008-05-14.
- o 88. "3rd Test Australia v England, match report". *Wisden*. 1938 edition. Retrieved 2007-08-22.
- o 89. "Laxman, Kumble in Wisden's top ten list". *Cricinfo*. 2001-07-26. Retrieved 2008-08-23.

- o 90. "The Ashes 4th Test Australia v England". *Wisden*. 1937 edition. Retrieved 2008-06-19.
- o 91. "5th Test Australia v England, match report". *Wisden*. 1938 edition. Retrieved 2007-08-22.
- o 92. "Test matches Winning a series after coming from behind". *Cricinfo*. Retrieved 2008-04-26.
- o 93. Wilfrid, Brookes (1939 edition). "The Australian team in England 1938". *Wisden*. Retrieved 2008-05-15.
- o 94. Kidd, Patrick (2006-05-09). "The hunt for 1,000". *The Times*. Retrieved 2008-08-23.
- o 95. "The Ashes, 1938, 1st Test". *Cricinfo*. Retrieved 2008-06-20.
- o 96. "2nd Test, 24 28 June 1938". *Cricinfo*. Retrieved 2008-05-14.
- o 97. "Third Test match: England v Australia 1938". *Wisden*. 1938 edition. Retrieved 2008-05-14.
- o 98. Bradman (1950), pp 115 118.
- o 99. "4th Test England v Australia, match report". *Wisden*. 1939 edition. Retrieved 2007-08-08.
- o 100. "5th Test England v Australia, match report". *Wisden*. 1939 edition. Retrieved 2007-08-22.
- o 101. Lynch, Steven (2004-04-12). "The highest score in Test cricket". *Cricinfo*. Retrieved 2008-08-23.
- o 102. Bradman (1950), p 108.
- o 103. "Largest margin of victory (by an innings)". *Cricinfo*. Retrieved 2007-12-05.
- o 104. "Football in the Age of Instability (transcript)". *Australian Broadcasting Corporation*. 2002-10-04. Retrieved 2008-08-23.
- o 105. "Hundreds in consecutive innings". *Cricinfo*. Retrieved 2008-08-23.
- o 106. Dunstan (1988), p 172.
- o 107. Williams (1996), pp 182 183. "Nevertheless, the Secretaryship of the Melbourne Cricket Club was, and indeed, still is one of the most attractive jobs in the world of Australian cricket ..."
- o 108. Coleman (1993) pp 425 426.
- o 109. Bradman (1950), p 120.
- o 1010. Harte (1993), pp 382 383.
- o 111. Williams (1996), p 187.
- o 112. Page (1983), p 266 267.
- o 113. Eason (2004), p 61.
- o 114. Bradman (1950), p 122.
- o 115. "Cricket: 'The Don' accused of underarm tactics in financial scandal". *New Zealand Herald*. 2001-11-24. Retrieved 2008-08-23.
- o 116. Hutchins, Brett. *Don Bradman: Challenging the Myth*. pp. 155 156. "The question within Adelaide business circles ever since has been whether Bradman, who was second in charge of the firm and Hodgetts' friend, had prior knowledge of the impending collapse. [These] ... dubious circumstances ... led to resentment towards Bradman among ... the Adelaide Exchange that is said to still linger today."
- o 117. Harte (1992), pp 392 393.
- o 118. Page (1983), pp 271 272.
- o 119. Bradman (1950), p 125.
- o 120. Eason (2004), p 337.

- 121. Williams (1996) pp 205 206. "It was all the more obvious that, on any analysis, the only figure of stature who could lead Australia back into the post-War cricket era was 'the little feller', the 'sick man of Adelaide', the wartime invalid now nearing forty. It is little wonder that all Australia wanted to know precisely what he was proposing to do."
- 122. "History from the maker". *Cricinfo*. Retrieved 2008-05-19.
- 123. Bradman (1950), p 126.
- 124. "1st Test Australia v England match report". *Wisden*. 1948 edition. Retrieved 2007-08-08.
- 125. Whitington (1974), p 190.
- 126. Fingleton (1949), p 22.
- 127. Bradman (1950), p 139.
- 128. "Australian XI v Indians at Sydney". *Cricinfo*. Retrieved 2008-05-15.
- 129. "First-class matches: Most hundreds in a career". *Records*. Cricinfo. Retrieved 2008-05-14. Bradman scored 117 centuries. At 14 May 2008, the closest Australians to the 100-century mark are Darren Lehmann and Justin Langer with 82. The other non-English players to score 100 centuries Viv Richards, Zaheer Abbas and Glenn Turner started their first-class cricket careers after Bradman had retired from all forms of cricket.
- 130. "Bradman and the Indian connection". *Cricinfo*. Retrieved 2008-08-23.
- 131. "Biographical essay by Michael Page". *State Library South Australia*. Retrieved 2008-05-19.
- 132. "Benaud rates Ponting's team alongside the Invincibles". *Cricinfo.com*. Retrieved 2008-08-23.
- 133. "Five Live's Greatest Team of all Time". *BBC*. Retrieved 2008-05-19.
- 134. Quoted by Page (1983), p 312.
- 135. "Sporting greats Australia reveres and treasures its sporting heroes.". *Australian Government Culture and Recreation Portal*. Retrieved 2008-08-23. "The 1948 Australian cricket team captained by Don Bradman, for example, became known as 'The Invincibles' for their unbeaten eight-month tour of England. This team is one of Australia's most cherished sporting legends."
- 136. Bradman (1950), p 152.
- 137. Robinson (1981), p 153.
- 138. It s an Honour: Knight Bachelor
- 139. Bradman Foundation Australia
- 140. Bradman (1950)
- 141. Perry (1995), p 569.
- 142. Williams (1996), p 251.
- 143. The following sources are, respectively, a Miller obituary from 2004, which lists Trumper and Bradman and a further piece from 2005, when Warne's portrait was added. Michael Atherton, the author of the second piece, curiously overlooks Trumper's portrait; other articles of the same period do similarly.
- 144. Selvey, Mike (2004-10-12). "Obituary: Keith Miller". *The Guardian*. Retrieved 2008-01-14.
- 145. Atherton, Michael. "Warne: still the incomparable master of spin bowler's craft". *The Telegraph*. Retrieved 2008-05-16.
- 146. "SCGT History". *Sydney Cricket & Sports Ground Trust*. Retrieved 2008-05-16.
- 147. "SACA Timeline". *South Australian Cricket Association*. Retrieved 2008-05-16.
- 148. Williams (1996), p 271.
- 149. "SACA History". *South Australian Cricket Association*. Retrieved 2008-05-16.

o 150. "Bradman Foundation". *Bradman Museum*. Archived from the original on 2007-08-31. Retrieved 2008-08-23.
o 151. It s an Honour: AC
o 152. Harte (1993), p 658.
o 153. Cashman (1996), p 58.
o 154. "Background: The 1960 61 West Indies tour of Australia". *Cricinfo*. Retrieved 2008-08-23.
o 155. "Cricket Australia: History". *Cricket Australia*. Retrieved 2008-08-23.
o 156. Page (1983), pp 350 355.
o 157. Eason (2004), p 15.
o 158. Harte (1993), p 587.
o 159. Haigh (1993), p 106.
o 160. Chappell, Ian; Mallett (2007). *Chappelli Speaks Out*. Ashley. Allen & Unwin. pp. 150. ISBN 1741750369.
o 161. Frith (2002), p 427.
o 162. "Sport Australia Hall of Fame History" at *sahof.org.au*
o 163. Williams (1996), p 274.
o 164. Eason (2004), p 16.
o 165. Eason (2004), p 65.
o 166. Eason (2004), p 73.
o 167. Eason (2004), p 67.
o 168. "Australian Cricket Hall of Fame Inductees". *Melbourne Cricket Ground*. Retrieved 2008-05-25.
o 169. "2000". *Wisden*. 2000 edition. Retrieved 2008-05-29.
o 170. Frith (2002), p 429.
o 171. "Bradman never missed a Tendulkar innings in last five years". *Cricinfo*. 2001-08-16. Retrieved 2008-08-23.
o 172. "Adelaide Oval". *The Bradman Trail*. Retrieved 2008-05-19.
o 173. *Bradman dies at 92*. BBC News. Retrieved on 14 May 2008
o 174. Hutchins (2002), p 4.
o 175. "Previous Australia Post Australian Legends". *Australia Post*. Retrieved 2008-04-26.
o 176. "Bradman coin among best in the world". *Royal Australian Mint*. 2002-10-22. Retrieved 2008-08-23.
o 177. Williams (1996), pp 78 79.
o 178. Eason (2004), p 55.
o 179. "The Bradman Trail". *The Bradman Trail*. Retrieved 2008-05-19.
o 180. "Question: What were the difficulties faced in Sir Donald Bradmans life?". *Bradman Museum*. Archived from the original on 2007-08-31. Retrieved 2008-08-23.
o 181. "Just a few tears as Miller's tale celebrated". *The Age*. Retrieved 2008-05-19.
o 182. "Death Of Sir Donald Bradman". *Parliament of New South Wales*. Retrieved 2008-05-19.
o 183. Eason (2004), p 56.
o 184. Wallace, (2004), Chapter 6.
o 185. "Bradman dies at 92". *BBC Sport*. 2001-02-26. Retrieved 2008-05-19.
o 186. "Bradman's son reclaims name". *CNN Sports Illustrated*. 2000-01-07. Retrieved 2008-08-23.
o 187. "Feeling pretty average? Slam down a Bradman". *smh.com.au*. Retrieved 2008-05-19.

○ 188. "PM Son warns of against Bradman worship". *ABC*. Retrieved 2008-05-19.

○ 189. Eason (2004), p 57.

○ 190. "Farewell to the Don". *Time*. Retrieved 2008-08-23.

○ 191. Bradman (1950), p 20.

○ 192. Eason (2004), p 88.

○ 193. Robinson (1981), p 139.

○ 194. Bradman (1950), p 74.

○ 195. Fingleton (1949), pp 209 211.

○ 196. "Market in Bradmanesque form". *www.capitalmarket.co.in*. 7 February 2007. Retrieved 2009-03-02.

○ 197. Perrin, Andrew (2004-10-04). "Asia's Heroes Muttiah Muralitharan". *Time*. Retrieved 2008-08-23.

○ 198. "Howard the Bradman of politics: Hockey". *ABC News*. 2007-09-13. Retrieved 2008-08-23.

○ 199. Eason (2004), p 184.

○ 200. Crook, Frank (2008-02-08). "Real life drama on TV". *The Daily Telegraph*. Retrieved 2008-06-24.

○ 201. "Our Don Bradman (music): a snappy fox trot song / by Jack O'Hagan". *Music Australia*. National Library of Australia. Retrieved 2008-05-20.

○ 202. "Bradman". *Dumb Things*. Retrieved 2008-05-20.

○ 203. "Greats attend Bradman tribute". *BBC Sport*. 2001-03-25. Retrieved 2008-08-23.

○ 204. "Dimensions transcript of interview with Kamahl". *Australia Broadcasting Corporation*. Retrieved 2008-06-17.

○ 205. "Corporations Amendment Regulations 2000 (No 8)". *Corporations Regulations 2001*. Retrieved 2008-06-17.

○ 206. "Corporations Regulations 2001". Retrieved 2008-06-17.

○ 207. "Statsguru DG Bradman Test matches Batting analysis". *Cricinfo*. Retrieved 2008-06-20.

○ 208. "Statsguru DG Bradman Test Bowling Bowling analysis". *Cricinfo*. Retrieved 2008-06-20.

○ 209. "Bradman's Career Statistics". *Bradman Museum*. Archived from the original on 2007-09-01. Retrieved 2008-08-23.

○ 2010. "Test matches: Highest career batting average". *Cricinfo*. Retrieved 2008-05-19. Players with a "Span" end date of 2008 are still playing Test cricket.

○ 211. "Test matches Batting records". *Cricinfo*. Retrieved 2008-05-17.

○ 212. "Players Batting 30 Innings with 10% Centuries". *Howstat*. Retrieved 2008-05-29.

○ 213. "Records Test matches Highest partnership for the fifth wicket". *Cricinfo*. Retrieved 2008-05-17.

○ 214. "Records Test matches Highest partnership for the sixth wicket". *Cricinfo*. Retrieved 2008-05-17.

○ 215. "Records Test matches Most runs in an innings (by batting position)". *Cricinfo*. Retrieved 2008-05-17.

○ 216. "Most runs against West Indies, and most wickets against anyone". *Cricinfo*. Retrieved 2008-05-17.

○ 217. "Records Test matches Most runs in a series". *Cricinfo*. Retrieved 2008-05-17.

○ 218. "Current Test Records still held by D.G. Bradman". *Bradman Museum*. Archived from the original on 2007-09-01. Retrieved 2008-08-23.

○ 219. "Records Test matches Most runs in a day". *Cricinfo*. Retrieved 2008-05-17.

○ 220. "DG Bradman Test matches All-round analysis". *Cricinfo*. Retrieved 2008-05-17.

o 221. "Test matches: Most double hundreds in a series". *Cricinfo*. Retrieved 2008-05-19.
o 222. "Test matches Batting records". *Cricinfo*. Retrieved 2008-05-17.
o 223. "Records Test matches Hundreds in consecutive matches". *Cricinfo*. Retrieved 2008-05-17.
o 224. "Fastest to 2000 Runs". *Cricinfo*. Retrieved 1 January 2010.
o 225. "Fastest to 3000 Runs". *Cricinfo*. Retrieved 1 January 2010.
o 226. "Fastest to 4000 Runs". *Cricinfo*. Retrieved 1 January 2010.
o 227. "Fastest to 5000 Runs". *Cricinfo*. Retrieved 1 January 2010.
o 228. "Fastest to 6000 Runs". *Cricinfo*. Retrieved 1 January 2010.
o 229. "Highest frequency of hundreds and fiver-fors". *Cricinfo*. Retrieved 2008-08-23.
o 230. "DG Bradman Test matches All-round analysis". *Cricinfo*. Retrieved 2008-05-17.
o 231. Buckley, Will (2007-09-16). "Ali? Laver? Best? No, the Williams sisters". *The Observer*. Retrieved 2008-08-23.
o 232. Shaw, John (2001-02-27). "Sir Donald Bradman, 92, Cricket Legend, Dies". *The New York Times*. Retrieved 2008-08-23.
o 233. Adams, Kathleen; et al. (2001-03-04). "Milestones". *Time*. Retrieved 2008-08-23.
o 234. *Six Giants of the Wisden Century* Neville Cardus, *Wisden Cricketers' Almanack*, 1963]. Retrieved on 8 November 2008.

References (URLs online)

o Bradman, Don (1950): *Farewell to Cricket*, 1988 Pavilion Library reprint. ISBN 1 85145 225 7.

o Cashman, Richard et al. editors (1996): *The Oxford Companion to Australian Cricket*, Oxford University Press. ISBN 0 19 553575 8.

o Coleman, Robert (1993): *Seasons In the Sun: the Story of the Victorian Cricket Association*, Hargreen Publishing Company. ISBN 0 949905 59 3.

o Davis, Charles (2000): *The Best Of the Best: A New Look at the Great Cricketers and Changing Times*, ABC Books. ISBN 0 733308 99 6.

o Dunstan, Keith (1988, rev. ed.): *The Paddock That Grew*, Hutchinson Australia. ISBN 0 09 169170 2.

o Eason, Alan (2004): *The A-Z of Bradman*, ABC Books. ISBN 0 7333 1517 8.

o Fingleton, Jack (1949): *Brightly Fades the Don*, 1985 Pavilion Library reprint. ISBN 0 907516 69 6.

o Frith, David (2002): *Bodyline Autopsy*, ABC Books. ISBN 0 7333 1321 3.

o Harte, Chris (1993): *A History of Australian Cricket*, Andre Deutsch. ISBN 0 233 98825 4.

o Haigh, Gideon. "Sir Donald Bradman at 100." *The Monthly*, August 2008.

o Haigh, Gideon (1993): *The Cricket War the Inside Story of Kerry Packer's World Series Cricket*, Text Publishing Company. ISBN 1 86372 027 8.

o Hutchins, Brett (2002): *Don Bradman: Challenging the Myth*, Cambridge University Press. ISBN 0 521 82384 6.

:

o O'Reilly, Bill (1985): *Tiger 60 Years of Cricket*, William Collins. ISBN 0 00 217477 4.

o McGilvray, Alan & Tasker, Norman (1985): *The Game Is Not the Same*, ABC Books. ISBN 9 780642 527387.

o Page, Michael (1983): *Bradman The Illustrated Biography*, Macmillan Australia. ISBN 0 333 35619 5.

o Perry, Roland (1995): *The Don A Biography of Sir Donald Bradman*, Macmillan. ISBN 0 73290827 2.

o Robinson, Ray (1981 rev. ed.): *On Top Down Under*, Cassell Australia. ISBN 0 7269 7281 5.

o Rosenwater, Irving (1978): *Sir Donald Bradman A Biography*, Batsford. ISBN 0 71 340664 X.

o Wallace, Christine (2004): *The Private Don*, Allen & Unwin. ISBN 9 78174175 1581.

o Whitington, RS (1974): *The Book of Australian Test Cricket 1877 1974*, Wren Publishing. ISBN 0 85885 197 0.

o Williams, Charles (1996): *Bradman: An Australian Hero*, 2001 Abacus reprint. ISBN 0 3491 1475 7.

o *Wisden Cricketers Almanack*: various editions, accessed at http://content-aus.cricinfo.com/wisdenalmanack/content/story/almanack/index.html

Websites (URLs online)

o Player Profile: Donald Bradman from Cricinfo
o Player Profile: Donald Bradman from CricketArchive
o Bradman Museum and Bradman Oval
o Bradman Digital Library State Library of South Australia
o The Bradman Trail
o Don Bradman on Picture Australia
o Interview with Bradman 1930

Sporting positions

- Preceded by **Vic Richardson**: **Australian Test cricket captains** 1936/7 1938: Succeeded by **Bill Brown**
- Preceded by **Bill Brown**: **Australian Test cricket captains** 1946/7 1948: Succeeded by **Lindsay Hassett**
- Preceded by **Bill Dowling**: **Chairman Australian Cricket Board** 1960 1963: Succeeded by **Ewart Macmillan**
- Preceded by **Bob Parish**: **Chairman Australian Cricket Board** 1969 1972: Succeeded by **Tim Caldwell**
- Records
- Preceded by **Andy Sandham**: **World Record Highest individual score in Test cricket** 334 vs England at Leeds 1930: Succeeded by **Wally Hammond**

A hyperlinked version of this chapter is at http://booksllc.net?q=Donald%5FBradman

INDEX